Student Nurse
Nutrition and Hydration

Survival Guide

Linda Field

First published 2010 by Pearson Education Limited

Published 2013 by Routledge
2 Park Square, Milton Park, Abingdon, Oxon OX14 4RN
711 Third Avenue, New York, NY 10017, USA

Routledge is an imprint of the Taylor & Francis Group, an informa business

Copyright © 2010, Taylor & Francis.

The right of Linda Field to be identified as author of this work has been asserted
by her in accordance with the Copyright, Designs and Patents Act 1988.

ISBN: 978-0-273-72871-9 (hbk)

British Library Cataloguing-in-Publication Data
A catalogue record for this book is available from the British Library

Library of Congress Cataloging-in-Publication Data
A catalog record for this book is available from the Library of Congress

Typeset in 8/9.5pt Helvetica by 35

contents

NUTRITION 3
  Nutritional requirements 3
  Nutritional needs 6
  Nutritional assessment 7
BODY MASS INDEX 8
  Waist circumference 9
FACTORS AFFECTING ABILITY TO EAT 9
  Physical 10
  Pathological 11
  Other 11
FACTORS INFLUENCING NUTRITION IN HOSPITAL 12
  Problems with the food 12
  Problems with the systems of supplying the food 12
CONSEQUENCES OF MALNUTRITION 13
  Feeding patients 14
  Other methods of feeding 16
WHEN SHOULD NUTRITIONAL SUPPORT BE CONSIDERED? 18
  Complications of nutritional support 19
HYDRATION 20
  Hydration requirements 20
  Regulation of body fluids 21
HORMONAL INFLUENCES 21
  Anti-diuretic hormone 21
  Renin 21
  Aldosterone 21
  Kidneys 22
ELECTROLYTES 22
FACTORS AFFECTING HYDRATION NEEDS 22
  Age 23
  Gender and body size 23
  Lifestyle 23
  Environmental temperature 23
  Pathology 24
  Diet 24
  Exercise 24
  Stress 24
FLUID IMBALANCES 25
  Hypervolaemia 25
  Hypovolaemia 25

METHODS OF ADMINISTRATION OF FLUIDS 26
    Oral 26
    Intravenous 27
    Subcutaneous 27
    Associated problems with intravenous and subcutaneous infusions 28
RECORDING FLUID BALANCE 28
    Accurate measurement of fluid intake 28
    Accurate measurement of fluid output 28
    Negative and positive fluid balance 29

Nutrition

■ NUTRITIONAL REQUIREMENTS

The body requires an adequate supply of **essential** nutrients to maintain health. These and their functions are listed below.

NUTRIENT	FUNCTION
Protein	Growth and repair, main constituent of hormones, enzymes and antibodies
Carbohydrates	Main source of energy
Fats	Source of energy; components of cell membranes; insulation
Vitamins	Helps body cells to function – only needed in small quantities
Minerals	Helps to maintain body functions e.g. calcium for bone growth and repair
Fibre	Helps to move food through the gastrointestinal tract
Salt	Provides the essential chemical elements for the body e.g. sodium and chloride

These **essential** nutrients must be present in a person's daily diet in variable amounts. It is important that a person consumes a 'balanced diet' of different types of foods containing proteins, carbohydrates and fats; this should also ensure the daily requirements of vitamins and minerals are taken.

There are guidelines for the recommended daily amounts (GDA) of these food groups. These are shown in the table below.

Guideline Daily Amounts (GDA)

	WOMEN	MEN	CHILDREN (5–10YRS)
Energy	2000 kcal	2500 kcal	1800 kcal
Protein	45 g	55 g	24 g
Carbohydrates of which **sugars** of which **starch**	230 g 90 g	300 g 120 g	220 g 85 g
Fat of which **saturates**	70 g 20 g	95 g 30 g	70 g 20 g
Fibre	24 g	24 g	15 g
Salt of which sodium	6 g 2.4 g	6 g 2.4 g	4 g 1.4 g

HINTS

You can see from the table above that both the GDA of sugars and saturated fat has been highlighted. Why do you think this is?

Too high an intake of sugars is not considered to be good for you. Sugars are high in calories and also contribute to dental decay and gum disease, particularly in children.

Saturated fats are considered to be 'bad' fats. Eating a lot of saturated fat increases the blood cholesterol level leading to damage to the cardiovascular system. Nutritionists recommend that only 10% of the daily calorie intake should come from saturated fats.

Daily intake of different food groups can sometimes be expressed as percentages (see chart below). This clearly indicates that, ideally, 55% of our daily food intake comes from carbohydrates, 30% from fats and 15% from proteins.

Proportion of daily intake of different food groups expressed as a percentage

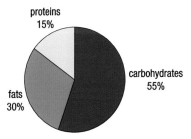

The body's energy requirements are chiefly met by carbohydrates, fats and proteins. Energy needs can differ from one person to another and are determined by:

1. The amount of energy needed to maintain involuntary body functions at rest, for example breathing production and secretion of hormones (basal metabolic rate BMR).
2. The amount of energy needed to metabolize food.
3. Physical activity.

Calorific value

The amount of energy that nutrients supply to the body is measured in calories. A **calorie (c, cal, kcal)** can be described as a unit of heat energy.

Different food types provide different amounts of calories.

- One gram of carbohydrate provides 4 kcals.
- One gram of protein provides 4 kcals.
- One gram of fat provides 9 kcals.
- One gram of alcohol provides 7 kcals.

■ NUTRITIONAL NEEDS

A person's nutritional needs can differ and are therefore not 'fixed in tablets of stone'. They can be influenced by a person's religious or cultural beliefs as indicated.

HINTS

What factors do you think may influence a healthy person's nutritional needs?

- Age.
- Culture.
- Gender.
- Pregnancy.
- Lifestyle.
- Amount of physical activity.
- Personal preference.
- Height and build.
- Religion.
- Financial situation.
- Knowledge about the nutritional value of different foods.

Special diets

Some people have an intolerance of certain food types and therefore have to consume a modified or 'special' diet.

For example, a gluten-free diet for people who suffer with Caeliac disease.

HINTS
You may wish to find out more about Coeliac disease.

Allergies
Certain foods, such as nuts, can bring about an allergic reaction when consumed by some people. Some of these reactions can be fatal if not treated immediately as they can cause **anaphylactic shock** to develop.

HINTS
You may wish to find out more about anaphylactic shock.

■ NUTRITIONAL ASSESSMENT

Nutritional assessment is carried out to identify patients who are 'at risk' of developing malnutrition and those who already have a poor nutritional status. It involves:

- Nutritional history.
- Nutritional screening.
- Recording physical measurements.

Nutritional history
This involves identifying what a person normally eats and will include such factors as likes and dislikes and cultural influences.

Nutritional screening
This involves identifying patients 'at risk' of malnutrition and those who are malnourished. This should be done on admission and continued on a weekly basis for patients in hospital as their condition may change. It can also be done

by the practice nurse in a GP setting if the patient is not in hospital.

Recording physical measurements

This includes weight, height (particularly in the children) body mass index and weight circumference.

HINTS

Patients who are identified as being 'moderate' to 'high risk' should be referred to the dietician for a more detailed assessment so a dietary plan can be implemented.

Body Mass Index (BMI)

A person's BMI is calculated by dividing the weight in kilograms by the square of the height in metres:

$$BMI = \frac{weight \ (kg)}{height \ (m)^2}$$

Calculate the BMI of a person who weighs 60kg and is 1.69m tall.

BMI measurements

BMI SCORE	INDICATION
Less than 20	Underweight
20–25	Normal healthy weight
25–29.9	Overweight
Over 30	Obese
Over 40	Very/morbidly obese

HINTS

The BMI can only be used on people over 18 years of age so is therefore unsuitable to assess children's weight.

The use of BMI does have limitations – it only measures body mass, not body fat. e.g. some athletes can have a high BMI but a relatively low body fat mass as they have an increased high lean muscle mass.

$$\text{Answer to BMI calculation} = \frac{60}{(1.69 \times 1.69)} = 21$$

■ WAIST CIRCUMFERENCE

This is a useful measurement with obese patients. It acts as an indicator of excess body fat and increased health risk.

HINTS

Men with a waist circumference of > 102 cm and women with a waist circumference of > 88 cm carry the same risk of developing cardiovascular disease as having a BMI of 30. This is because waist circumference is a measure of visceral or abdominal fat mass and is independent of height and muscle mass. Therefore, waist circumference is a useful indicator of excess body fat and increased health risk.

Reference / Lean, M. (1998) in Campbell, I. and Haslam, D. *Obesity: Your Questions Answered*, London: Churchill Livingstone, p.6.

Factors affecting ability to eat

Below are some factors that can be associated with the risk of malnutrition.

■ PHYSICAL

Is the person able to physically feed themselves?

HINTS

What sort of physical problems could affect a person's ability to eat?

There may be problems with dexterity if a person suffers with arthritis. They may have suffered a stroke and are unable to move one hand. There may be visual problems which will interfere with a person locating food if it is left on a locker.

Does the person suffer with difficulty in swallowing (dysphagia)?

HINTS

How would you recognise/detect this problem?

The person may be coughing or even choking as they are at risk of aspiration. They might be exhibiting signs of respiratory wheeze or gurgling. They may be drooling and have watery eyes.

Reference / Field, L. and Smith, B. (2008) *Nursing Care: an Essential Guide*, London: Pearson Education.

Does the person have any dental problems?

HINTS

How would you recognise/detect this problem?

The person may be reluctant to eat certain types of food that are quite hard or crunchy and require a lot of chewing. They may be wearing ill-fitting dentures that will contribute to difficulty with chewing. They may not wear any dentures.

You may be able to find this out when helping a person with personal hygiene and oral care.

■ PATHOLOGICAL

Certain kinds of conditions could affect a person's ability to eat. Some are listed below.

- **Mental condition** – depression/dementia.
- **Digestive tract functioning** – nausea, vomiting, pain, gastrointestinal (GI) surgery, GI diseases e.g. Crohn's disease, intestinal obstruction.
- **Neurological conditions** – multiple sclerosis, Parkinson's disease.
- **Major trauma** – patients are at greater risk of malnutrition following surgery for major trauma.
- **Malignant disease** – cancer is associated with weight loss particularly when the GI tract is involved.

■ OTHER

Other factors contributing to the risk of malnutrition are:

- **Certain medications** such as some types of analgesia i.e. opiates are associated with unpleasant side effects such as nausea and vomiting which can lead to anorexia (not to be confused with anorexia nervosa).
- **Nil-by-mouth regimes** can lead to patients not having access to food for several hours as most fasting regimes are not tailored for individual patients or the timing of their procedures.
- **Older patients** are at greater risk of malnutrition as their decreased lean body mass and other factors can compromise nutritional and fluid intake.
- **Socioeconomic factors** such as geographical location can affect access to shops, and increasing frailty in the

elderly may contribute to difficulties preparing food and cooking meals. Poverty and deprivation in any age group can lead to the development of malnutrition.

Factors influencing nutrition in hospital

Several factors can have an impact on hospital food and these are outlined below.

■ PROBLEMS WITH THE FOOD

HINTS

What do you think these problems may include? Think about a patient you may have visited in hospital and what were their comments on the food. Have you personal experience of hospital food? You may have come up with some of the issues outlined in the box below.

Problems with the food in hospital
- Poor quality
- Poor quantity
- Lack of variety
- Poor general appearance (bland and unappetising)
- Inappropriate timing

■ PROBLEMS WITH THE SYSTEMS OF SUPPLYING THE FOOD

HINTS

What do think these problems may include? Have you experienced any in practice when giving food to patients? Some of the issues related to supply of hospital food are identified below.

Problems with the systems of supplying food
- Inadequate budget spent on patients' food
- Poor monitoring of whether patients get appropriate food choices
- Poor positioning of food, so patient cannot reach their meals
- No system for monitoring and reporting whether food has been eaten
- Lack of responsibility for taking action when patients do not eat their meals
- Timing of food availability
- Gaining access to special foods and meals that people enjoy when ill
- Staff removing meals before patients have had a chance to eat
- Completion of menu sheets

Consequences of malnutrition

What do you think might be the effects of malnutrition on a patient? Think about a patient you have nursed who was malnourished.

Malnutrition has both economic and clinical risks. The risk of mortality is doubled in hospital patients and tripled in older people, both in hospital and following discharge.

Reference / Stratton and Elia (2007) in Shepherd, A. (2009) *Nutrition support 1: risk factors, causes and physiology of malnutrition*, Nursing Times, 105(4), 18–20.

Some of the main complications found in malnourished people are identified below.

Complications of malnutrition
- Delayed recovery
- Impaired immunity leading to sepsis
- Impaired wound healing
- Impaired gastrointestinal tract function
- Muscle atrophy
- Impaired cardiac function
- Impaired respiratory function
- Reduced renal function
- Apathy, depression
- Impaired psychosocial functioning
- Altered sleep patterns
- Impaired thermoregulation, increasing risk of hypothermia
- Atrophic skin, leading to pressure ulcers

Sources: National Patient Safety Agency (2008); Stratton *et al.* (2003); McWhirter and Pennington (1994).

It is estimated that malnutrition alone costs the NHS £7.3 billion annually.

Reference / Stratton and Elia (2007) in Shepherd, A. (2009) *Nutrition support 1: risk factors, causes and physiology of malnutrition*, Nursing Times, 105(4), 18–20.

■ FEEDING PATIENTS

Patients can be fed either orally, enterally or parentally. Below is the procedure involved when feeding an adult patient orally.

Reference / Nicol et al (2004) *Essential Nursing Skills*, London: Mosby.

Procedure

1. Find out what the patient would like to eat and drink and ensure there are no dietary restrictions or food allergies.
2. Ensure the patient is comfortable i.e. has an empty bladder, clean hands, clean mouth and, where relevant, clean dentures.
3. Ask/assist the patient to sit upright if their condition allows.
4. Check the patient is able to swallow – this will prevent choking and aspiration into the lungs.
5. Clear a space for the patient's tray.
6. Position a chair beside the bed for you to feed the patient.
7. Wash and dry your hands thoroughly before commencing feeding.
8. Wear an apron of the appropriate colour, according to local policy.
9. Protect the patient's clothing with a napkin or paper towel.
10. The patient may need assistance to cut up their food.
11. Tailor the speed and manner in which food/drink is offered according to the patient's needs/wishes. Do not hurry the patient.
12. Allow the patient time to chew and swallow the food before presenting the next mouthful.
13. Avoid asking questions while the patient is eating.
14. Respect the patient's dignity and use a napkin to remove any dribbles of food or drink that may run down the chin.
15. Encourage the patient to eat and drink if necessary but do not force the patient to eat once they have indicated they have had enough. Small amounts taken more frequently can be more successful.
16. After eating assist the patient to meet hygiene needs i.e. mouth, teeth and hands.

17. Remove apron and wash hands.
18. Ensure food and drink taken are recorded on the appropriate chart.
19. Report any food refusal or vomiting to the nurse in charge.

■ OTHER METHODS OF FEEDING

Enteral feeding

This involves the giving of nutrients in fluid form via the gastrointestinal tract either via the nose (naso-gastric), stomach (gastrostomy) or jejunum (jejunostomy). Enteral feeding can also include the giving of fortified foods, snacks and oral nutritional supplements.

Naso-gastric feeding

This involves the insertion of a naso-gastric tube into one of the patient's nostrils which is then passed into the nasopharynx, oropharynx and into the alimentary tract reaching the stomach. Naso-gastric tubes are used on patients who have intact cough and gag reflexes, who have adequate gastric emptying and who require short-term feeding i.e. less than six weeks.

Gastrostomy and jejunostomy

These enteral devices are used for more long-term nutritional support and are used for usually more than 6 to 8 weeks. The tubes are passed surgically by laparoscopy through the abdominal wall into the stomach (gastrostomy) or into the jejunum (jejunostomy). The surgical opening is sutured tightly around the tube or catheter to prevent leakage. They are often referred to as a **percutaneous endoscopic gastrostomy (PEG)** or **percutaneous endoscopic jejunostomy (PEJ)**.

Position of a percutaneous endoscopic gastrostomy in the stomach

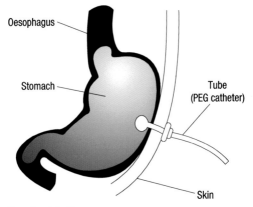

Parenteral feeding

Parenteral nutrition (PN) is used when the gastrointestinal (GI) tract cannot be used as there is an interruption in the continuity of the GI tract. Sometimes referred to as **Total parenteral nutrition (TPN)**, it involves the giving of solutions of dextrose, water, fat, proteins, electrolytes, vitamins and trace elements intravenously. TPN will be used for patients who are severely nutritionally compromised.

HINTS

What type of conditions would lead a patient to be severely nutritionally compromised? Try to think about a patient you have nursed who was receiving TPN.

NICE guidelines on nutrition (2006) recommend that parenteral feeding should be used in adults who are malnourished or who are at risk of this in the clinical situations shown in the box below.

Reasons for using parenteral feeding
- Patients with inadequate or unsafe oral and/or enteral nutrition intake
- Any person with a non-functional, inaccessible or perforated (leaking) GI tract

---

The GI route is the preferred route for nutritional support due to the lower risk of infection. PN should be limited to patients with intestinal failure, fistula, paralytic ileus and bowel obstruction. Infection control is vital when caring for a patient receiving TPN due to the higher risk of infection.

When should nutritional support be considered?

According to the NICE guidelines on nutrition (2006) nutritional support should be considered for the following patients:
1. Patients with a BMI < 18.5.
2. Unintentional weight loss > 10% over the past 3–6 months.
3. BMI < 20 and unintentional weight loss > 5% over the past 3–6 months.
4. Those who have eaten little or nothing for more than five days and who are unlikely to eat for the next five days or longer.

5. Patients with poor gastrointestinal (GI) absorption, high nutrient losses or increased nutritional needs.

Reference / National Institute for Clinical Excellence (2006) *Nutritional support in adults: oral nutrition support, enteral tube feeding and parenteral nutrition*, London: NICE, www.nice.org.uk/guidance/CG32.

■ COMPLICATIONS OF NUTRITIONAL SUPPORT

Refeeding syndrome

Before commencing tube feeding the degree of malnourishment should be assessed. Refeeding syndrome is a potentially lethal condition that can occur in acutely ill or severely malnourished patients who are given glucose solutions or other forms of enteral/parenteral nutrition too quickly.

Common signs are:

- low plasma levels of potassium, phosphate, magnesium and thiamine.
- salt and water retention.
- electrolyte imbalances, if untreated, can lead to cardiac, respiratory, hepatic and neuromuscular system disorders leading to clinical complications and death.

NICE (2006) suggests enteral nutrition support should be introduced cautiously in seriously ill or injured people, commencing with only 50% of total energy and protein requirements, which should build up to 100% over 24–48 hours depending on urea and electrolyte tests and clinical monitoring.

Reference / National Institute for Clinical Excellence (2006) *Nutritional support in adults: oral nutrition support, enteral tube feeding and parenteral nutrition*, London: NICE, www.nice.org.uk/guidance/CG32.

Monitoring nutritional intake

It is vitally important that all amounts of food eaten are recorded on a nutritional chart. The patient should be weighed weekly (if possible) and any weight loss or gain recorded on the nutritional chart and documented in the patient's notes. This ensures that an up-to-date record is kept of the patient's nutritional status and any changes needed e.g. extra nutritional supplements can be implemented. If a visit from the dietician is warranted then all information is available.

Hydration

■ HYDRATION REQUIREMENTS

The body requires fluid intake and output to be finely balanced.

HINTS

Why is it important that an accurate fluid balance is maintained? A delicate balance of fluid and electrolyte levels is needed in order to allow all bodily activities to occur. Fluid balance is regulated by fluid intake and output and hormonal influences.

Normal daily average fluid intake and output

FLUID INTAKE		FLUID OUTPUT		
Drink	1500	Urine	1500	
Food	750	Insensible Loss:	Lungs	400
Food metabolism	250		Skin	350
		Sweat	100	
		Faeces	200	

■ REGULATION OF BODY FLUIDS

The amount and volume of fluids in the body is finely tuned and needs to remain constant. This process is influenced by fluid intake and fluid output, hormonal and kidney activity.

HINTS

Do you know which hormones have an influence on fluid balance? These are discussed below.

Hormonal influences

■ ANTI-DIURETIC HORMONE (ADH)

ADH is produced by the hypothalamus and released from the posterior pituitary gland at the base of the brain. Its action is to **increase water reabsorption** via the kidneys. ADH is released when there is a reduction in fluid in the body e.g. haemorrhage, severe vomiting and diarrhoea.

■ RENIN

Renin is secreted from the kidneys when blood flow through the kidneys is reduced. Renin converts inactive angiotensinogen into angiotensin 11, which acts by narrowing the blood vessels in the kidney – this increases the blood pressure and raises the blood flow through the kidneys.

■ ALDOSTERONE

This hormone is secreted by the adrenal cortex and the main action of aldosterone is to regulate the reabsorption of sodium and water.

■ KIDNEYS

The kidneys regulate the amount of water reabsorbed back into the body. If the body loses excess fluid the kidneys will conserve water, conversely, if there is too much fluid in the body the kidneys will reabsorb less water.

Electrolytes

Electrolytes are transported through the body in water, so any fluid imbalance results in an electrolyte imbalance. **Electrolytes are charged ions capable of conducting electricity.** They carry either a positive or negative charge. They are present in all body fluids and fluid compartments. There is an equal balance of positively charged ions (cations) and negatively charged ions (anions). Electrolytes perform several important functions including:

1. Maintaining fluid balance
2. Contributing to acid-base regulation
3. Facilitating enzyme reactions
4. Transmitting neuromuscular reactions

Factors affecting hydration needs

HINTS

What factors do you think may alter a patient's hydration needs? How may these factors interfere with the finely tuned fluid balance in the body?

Think about patients you have nursed who required more or less fluids.

■ AGE

Infants and children have a quicker fluid turnover due to increased fluid loss from metabolic processes. They also have immature kidneys which contributes to the increased fluid loss.

In the older person the thirst response can be reduced and the kidneys may be less able to conserve water; this can increase the **risk of dehydration** in this age group.

■ GENDER AND BODY SIZE

Water accounts for 46–60% of the average adult's weight, however, females have more body fat and less body water than males. Males have more lean tissue and therefore hold more water. Body size also has an effect e.g. an obese person has even less lean tissue and water accounts for only 30–40% of total body weight.

■ LIFESTYLE

What a person eats and drinks can affect fluid and electrolyte balance e.g. if a person is malnourished or has an eating disorder. Stress also has an effect on cell metabolism and stress hormones, such as adrenaline, reduce urine output leading to an increase in blood volume.

■ ENVIRONMENTAL TEMPERATURE

Fluid is lost through sweating when in a hot environment and during strenuous exercise. Both salt and water are lost and can quickly lead to depletion if not replaced. There is also insensible loss through increased respiration.

■ PATHOLOGY

There are many diseases and conditions that can affect a person's fluid balance. Some of these are listed below:

1. Congestive cardiac failure
2. Renal failure
3. Liver cirrhosis
4. Pregnancy
5. Brain damage
6. Over-infusion of intravenous fluids
7. Haemorrhage
8. Trauma
9. Gastrointestinal problems
10. Diabetes mellitus

■ DIET

Diet can affect fluid and electrolyte imbalance. For example, people with eating disorders or who are malnourished may be deficient in fluids and electrolytes.

■ EXERCISE

Exercise promotes calcium balance reducing the risk of osteoporosis in older people.

■ STRESS

Stress can increase cellular metabolism and certain stress hormones, for example, adrenaline, decrease urine output resulting in an overall increase in blood volume.

Fluid imbalances

The balance between hypervolaemia and hypovolaemia

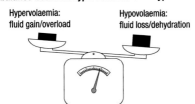

Hypervolaemia:
fluid gain/overload

Hypovolaemia:
fluid loss/dehydration

■ HYPERVOLAEMIA

Hypervolaemia is the term used to describe fluid overload. This basically means there is too much fluid in the body. There are three main causes for fluid volume excess. These are:

1. Excess fluid intake
2. Excess sodium intake
3. Failure of regulatory mechanisms

■ HYPOVOLAEMIA

Hypovolaemia denotes lack of fluid in the body and is very often described as '**dehydration**'.

HINTS

How would you recognise a person was suffering with hypervolaemia?

What signs and symptoms would they present with?

What about if a person was dehydrated: how would they present?

The following table summarises these clinical signs and symptoms.

OBSERVATION	FLUID DEPLETION	FLUID OVERLOAD
Weight	Loss	Gain
Blood pressure	Lowered	Normal or raised
Respiration	Rapid and shallow	Rapid, moist cough
Pulse	Rapid, weak and thready	Rapid
Urine output	Reduced and concentrated	Increased or decreased
Skin	Dry, less elastic	Oedematous
Saliva	Thick and viscous	Copious and frothy
Tongue	Dry and coated	Moist
Thirst	Present	No disturbance
Face	Sunken eyes (severe depletion)	Peri-orbital oedema
Temperature	May be raised	No disturbance

Reference / Place and Field (1997) *The Management of Fluid Balance*, Nursing Times, 93, 46–48.

Methods of administration of fluids

HINTS

What methods of administration of fluids have you seen when in practice? These are discussed below.

■ ORAL

This is the commonest route and used for most patients. It is important to ensure the patient does not suffer with dysphagia as they can be at risk of aspiration which could develop into pneumonia if not detected.

■ INTRAVENOUS

Fluid can be given directly into the vein through a cannula. It is extremely important that 'strict **asepsis**' is maintained during the infusion and that the amount of fluid infused is calculated to ensure the circulatory system is not overloaded and that an adequate fluid balance is maintained.

HINTS

How is the amount of fluid infused calculated? There is a formula you can follow when calculating the rate at which the infusion should be set to ensure the patient receives the prescribed amount of intravenous fluid.

$$\text{Rate (drops per minute)} = \frac{\text{volume to be infused}}{\text{time in hours}} \times \frac{\text{drop rate}}{60 \text{ minutes}}$$

The drop rate is found on the drip set packaging and is usually 20 drops/minute.

EXAMPLE

500 mls of normal saline to be infused in 4 hours (the drop rate is 20)

$$\frac{500}{4} \times \frac{20}{60} = \frac{500 \times 20}{240} = 41.6 = 42 \text{ drops/min}$$

■ SUBCUTANEOUS

With this method fluid is infused into the subcutaneous layer which lies directly under the skin. It is important to observe the cannulation site for any signs of infection.

■ ASSOCIATED PROBLEMS WITH INTRAVENOUS AND SUBCUTANEOUS INFUSIONS

HINTS

Problems or complications can occur with intravenous and subcutaneous infusions. These include:

1. Leakage of fluid around the cannula site
2. The intravenous administration or 'giving' set can become blocked
3. Extravasation – this is when fluid leaks from the vein into the interstitial fluid, sometimes referred to as 'tissuing'
4. Infection – this can occur around the cannula site and can give rise to inflammation of the vein – **phlebitis**

Recording fluid balance

■ ACCURATE MEASUREMENT OF FLUID INTAKE

It is vital that a patient's fluid intake is accurately recorded so the doctor, nurse and other members of the healthcare team can make an accurate assessment of how much fluid the patient has had. This can influence any treatment or medication prescribed.

■ ACCURATE MEASUREMENT OF FLUID OUTPUT

It is also extremely important that all fluid lost from the body is recorded accurately to give a clear picture of the patient's fluid balance. This includes fluid loss through urine by continuous bladder drainage from a catheter or urine collected in a bed pan if the patient can void naturally, plus 'insensible' loss through lungs, skin, sweat and faeces.

■ NEGATIVE AND POSITIVE FLUID BALANCE

A patient's fluid balance can be calculated from the amount of fluid taken in balanced with the amount of fluid lost from the body.

HINTS

If a patient has taken in 2540 mls of fluid and the output is 1799 mls is this person in negative or positive balance?

Negative balance

This occurs when the fluid input is less than the fluid output and the patient is 'at risk' of developing dehydration.

Positive balance

When the patient's fluid input is more than the patient's fluid output the patient is said to have a positive fluid balance.

Answer to activity:

the patient's fluid input is	2540 mls
the patient's fluid output is	1799 mls
positive balance of	741 mls

When completing fluid balance charts it is worth taking note of the tips outlined below:

Tips on recording fluid balance charts

1. Make sure both the patient and staff know the patient is on a fluid balance chart and that all fluid input and output needs to be recorded on the fluid balance chart
2. Always check with the patient when updating the fluid balance chart
3. If output is > input, the patient has a negative fluid balance
4. If input is > output the patient is in a positive fluid balance
5. Positive or negative balances of greater then 500 mls should be reported
6. Urine output should be approximately 30 mls/hr: if urine output is < 30 mls/hr report to the nurse in charge
7. Gain or loss of 1 kg of body weight equates to 1 litre of fluid retained or lost

---

Shift roster

DAY	DATE	SHIFT
MONDAY		
TUESDAY		
WEDNESDAY		
THURSDAY		
FRIDAY		
SATURDAY		
SUNDAY		